PARASITES WITHIN

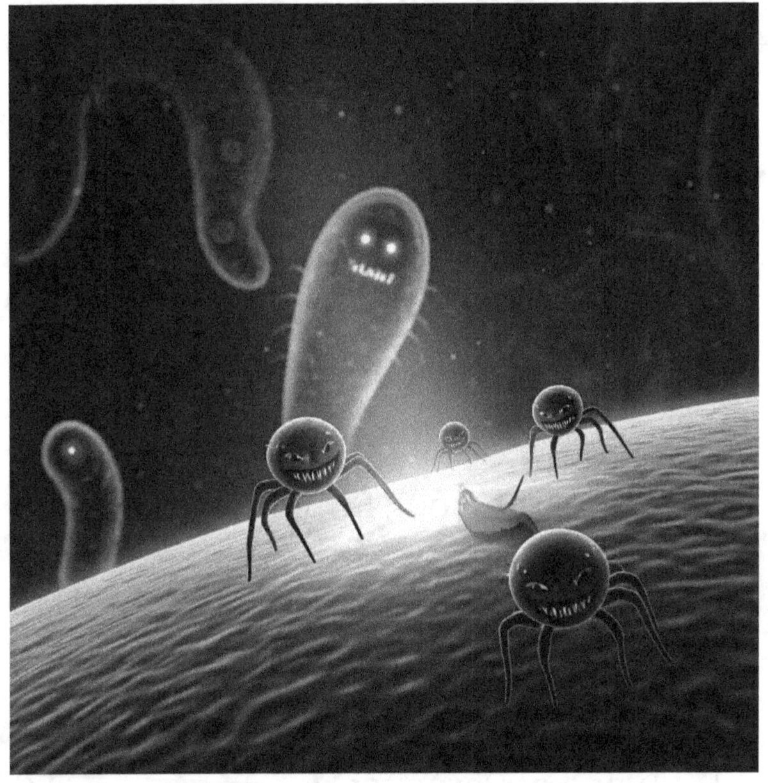

THE COMPLEX INTERPLAY BETWEEN HUMANS AND THEIR INVISIBLE MICROBIAL INVADERS

By Robert Anderson Love Wins

http://RobertAndersonLoveWins.com

TABLE OF CONTENTS

Intentions:

1. **Educate and Inform:** To provide readers with a comprehensive understanding of the diverse world of parasites, their life cycles, and their impact on human health.

2. **Promote Public Health Awareness:** To highlight the importance of preventive measures, such as proper hygiene, sanitation, and vector control, in reducing the burden of parasitic diseases.

3. **Foster Scientific Curiosity:** To inspire readers to delve deeper into the fascinating field of parasitology and contribute to scientific research.

4. **Encourage Global Health Initiatives:** To advocate for increased funding and support for global health programs aimed at

combating parasitic diseases, particularly in resource-limited settings.

The vision of "Parasites Within" is to empower readers with knowledge and inspire action. By understanding the intricate relationship between humans and parasites, readers can become informed advocates for public health and contribute to efforts to eradicate parasitic diseases.

Ultimately, this book aims to inspire a new generation of scientists, healthcare professionals, and global citizens to work together to create a healthier world, free from the burden of parasitic infections.

Imagine a world teeming with life, not just the life we see with the naked eye, but a microscopic universe of organisms, many of which have evolved to rely on us for their survival. These unseen invaders, known as parasites, have coexisted with humans for millennia, shaping our history, health, and even our behavior.

From the tiny tapeworm winding its way through our intestines to the elusive malaria parasite lurking within our blood cells, these organisms have developed intricate strategies to exploit our bodies. Some are benign, causing little to no harm, while others can cause debilitating diseases, even death.

IMPORTANCE OF UNDERSTANDING HOST-PARASITE INTERACTIONS

Understanding the complex relationship between humans and parasites is crucial for several reasons:

Public Health: By studying parasite biology and transmission, we can develop effective strategies to prevent and control parasitic infections.

Drug Discovery: Understanding the molecular mechanisms of parasite infection can lead to the development of new drugs and treatments.

Evolutionary Biology: Parasites have played a significant role in shaping human evolution, influencing our immune systems and genetic makeup.

Ecological Balance: Parasites play a vital role in ecosystems, regulating populations and influencing food webs.

In the following chapters, we will delve into the fascinating world of parasites, exploring their diversity, life cycles, and impact on human health. We will examine the intricate strategies that parasites employ to infect their hosts, evade the immune system, and reproduce. We will also discuss the various ways in which humans have adapted to coexist with these parasites, developing immune defenses and cultural practices to minimize their impact.

By the end of this book, you will have a deeper understanding of the complex and often surprising world of parasites. You will appreciate the delicate balance between host and parasite, and you will gain a new perspective on the interconnectedness of all living things.

1.1 DEFINITION AND CLASSIFICATION OF PARASITES

A parasite is an organism that lives on or in another organism, known as a host, deriving nourishment from it without providing any benefit in return. This parasitic relationship can be beneficial to the parasite but often detrimental to the host.

Parasites can be classified into two main groups:

1.2 TYPES OF PARASITES

1.2.1 ECTOPARASITES

Ectoparasites live on the external surface of their host. They often have specialized structures for attachment, such as claws, hooks, or suckers. Common examples of ectoparasites include:

Lice: Small, wingless insects that feed on human blood.

Mites: Tiny arachnids that can infest the skin, causing various skin conditions.

Ticks: Blood-sucking arachnids that can transmit diseases like Lyme disease.

1.2.2 ENDOPARASITES

Endoparasites live within the body of their host. They can inhabit various organs and tissues, including the digestive tract, lungs, blood, and brain. Common examples of endoparasites include:

Protozoa: Single-celled organisms that can cause diseases like malaria, amoebiasis, and giardiasis.

1.3 LIFE CYCLES AND TRANSMISSION MECHANISMS

Parasites have complex life cycles that often involve multiple hosts. These life cycles can vary widely, but they typically involve the following stages:

Infective Stage: The stage at which the parasite is capable of infecting a new host.

Developmental Stage: The stage during which the parasite grows and matures within the host.

Reproductive Stage: The stage at which the parasite reproduces, producing offspring that can infect new hosts.

Parasites are transmitted to their hosts through various mechanisms, including:

Direct Contact: Physical contact with an infected person or animal, such as through skin-to-skin contact or sexual transmission.

Indirect Contact: Contact with contaminated objects, such as clothing, bedding, or toys.

Vector-Borne Transmission: Transmission through the bite of an infected arthropod, such as a mosquito, tick, or flea.

Ingestion: Ingestion of contaminated food or water.

1.4 Host Specificity and Adaptations

Parasites have evolved various adaptations to survive and reproduce within their hosts. These adaptations include:

Host Specificity: Many parasites are highly specific to certain host species. This specificity is often determined by the parasite's ability to recognize and attach to specific host tissues.

Immune Evasion: Parasites have developed strategies to evade the host's immune system, such as producing molecules that mimic host proteins or suppressing the host's immune response.

Nutrient Acquisition: Parasites have evolved specialized structures to efficiently acquire nutrients from their host. For example, tapeworms have a complex digestive system that allows them to absorb nutrients directly from the host's intestine.

By understanding the diversity, life cycles, and adaptations of parasites, we can develop effective strategies to prevent and control parasitic infections and protect public health.

THE MEDICAL AND PUBLIC HEALTH SIGNIFICANCE OF ECTOPARASITES AND ENDOPARASITES

While ectoparasites like lice, mites, and ticks may cause discomfort, itching, and skin irritation, their primary public health significance lies in their potential to transmit serious diseases. For instance:

Ticks: Can transmit Lyme disease, Rocky Mountain spotted fever, and other tick-borne illnesses.

Mites: Can cause scabies, a highly contagious skin infestation.

Lice: While typically a nuisance, head lice can cause discomfort and social stigma.

ENDOPARASITES

Endoparasites pose a more significant threat to global health, especially in developing countries. They can cause a wide range of diseases, leading to severe morbidity and mortality. Some notable examples include:

HELMINTHS:

Intestinal worms: Can cause malnutrition, anemia, and growth retardation in children.

Schistosomiasis: A chronic disease affecting millions worldwide, causing liver, kidney, and bladder damage.

Filariasis: A debilitating disease that can lead to elephantiasis and other severe complications.

PROTOZOA:

Malaria: A life-threatening disease transmitted by mosquitoes, causing fever, chills, and potentially fatal complications.

Amoebiasis: A diarrheal disease that can lead to severe intestinal inflammation and, in some cases, liver abscesses.

Giardiasis: A common intestinal infection causing diarrhea, abdominal cramps, and fatigue.

These parasites contribute to poverty, malnutrition, and reduced productivity, particularly in regions with poor sanitation and inadequate healthcare. Therefore, understanding their biology, transmission, and control is crucial for global health initiatives.

CHAPTER 2: THE HUMAN IMMUNE SYSTEM: A DOUBLE-EDGED SWORD

2.1 OVERVIEW OF THE IMMUNE SYSTEM

The human immune system is a complex network of cells, tissues, and organs that work together to protect the body from infection.1 It consists of two main components: the innate immune system and the adaptive immune system.

2.2 IMMUNE RESPONSE TO PARASITIC INFECTIONS

2.2.1 INNATE IMMUNITY

The innate immune system provides a rapid, non-specific response to infection. It involves physical barriers, such as the skin and mucous membranes, as well as cellular and molecular defenses, such as phagocytic cells and inflammatory cytokines. In the case of parasitic infections, innate immunity can help to limit the spread of parasites and reduce the severity of disease.

2.2.2 ADAPTIVE IMMUNITY

The adaptive immune system provides a more specific and long-lasting response to infection. It involves the production of antibodies and the activation of T cells, which can recognize and eliminate specific pathogens. When a parasite infects the body, the adaptive immune system can generate a targeted response, leading to the production of antibodies that can neutralize the parasite or mark it for destruction by other immune cells.

2.3 IMMUNE EVASION STRATEGIES EMPLOYED BY PARASITES

Parasites have evolved a variety of strategies to evade the human immune system:

2.3.1 ANTIGENIC VARIATION

Many parasites can change their surface antigens, making it difficult for the immune system to recognize and eliminate them. This process, known as antigenic variation, allows parasites to persist in the host for extended periods.

2.3.2 IMMUNOSUPPRESSION

Some parasites can suppress the host's immune response, making it more difficult for the body to fight off infection. This can be achieved through a variety of mechanisms, such as producing immunosuppressive molecules or directly targeting immune cells.

By understanding the intricate interplay between the human immune system and parasitic organisms, we can develop more effective strategies to combat parasitic infections and protect public health.

CHAPTER 3: THE NEUROBIOLOGY OF PARASITISM

3.1 INTRODUCTION TO NEUROPARASITOLOGY

Neuroparasitology is an emerging field that explores the intricate relationship between parasites and the nervous systems of their hosts. Some parasites have evolved remarkable abilities to manipulate the behavior of their hosts, often to their own advantage.

3.2 PARASITES THAT MANIPULATE HOST BEHAVIOR

3.2.1 TOXOPLASMA GONDII: THE MIND MANIPULATOR

Toxoplasma gondii is a ubiquitous parasite that can infect a wide range of animals, including humans. In humans, it typically causes mild flu-like symptoms. However, in rodents, it can induce dramatic behavioral changes. Infected rodents become less fearful of cats, increasing their chances of being eaten by the parasite's definitive host. This manipulation is thought to be mediated by alterations in the neurotransmitter dopamine.

3.2.2 DICROCOELIUM DENDRITICUM: THE ZOMBIE ANT FUNGUS

Dicrocoelium dendriticum is a liver fluke that infects ants. It manipulates the ant's behavior, causing it to climb to the top of a blade of grass and clamp onto it with its mandibles. This behavior increases the likelihood that the ant will be eaten by a grazing animal, the parasite's definitive host.

3.3 MECHANISMS OF NEUROLOGICAL MANIPULATION

Parasites employ a variety of mechanisms to manipulate the behavior of their hosts:

3.3.1 NEUROTRANSMITTER MODULATION

Parasites can alter the levels of neurotransmitters in the host's brain, leading to changes in behavior and physiology. For example, Toxoplasma gondii can increase dopamine levels in the brains of infected rodents.

3.3.2 HOST BRAIN STRUCTURE ALTERATION

Some parasites can induce physical changes in the host's brain, such as the formation of cysts or tumors. These structural alterations can disrupt normal brain function and lead to behavioral changes.

3.4 THE ROLE OF THE GUT-BRAIN AXIS IN PARASITIC INFECTIONS

The gut-brain axis is a bidirectional communication pathway between the gastrointestinal tract and the central nervous system.1 Parasites that infect the gut can influence the gut microbiota, which in turn can affect brain function and behavior. This suggests that the gut may be a key target for parasitic manipulation.

Understanding the neurobiological mechanisms underlying parasitic manipulation can provide valuable insights into the evolution of host-parasite interactions and may lead to the development of new strategies to combat parasitic diseases.

4.1 COMMON PARASITIC INFECTIONS

Parasitic infections can have significant impacts on human health, ranging from mild discomfort to life-threatening diseases. Some of the most common parasitic infections include:

4.1.1 MALARIA

Malaria, caused by Plasmodium parasites, is a serious and sometimes fatal disease transmitted by the bite of an infected mosquito. Symptoms of malaria include fever, chills, headache, muscle aches, fatigue, nausea, and vomiting.

4.1.2 GIARDIASIS

Giardiasis is a diarrheal illness caused by the parasite Giardia intestinalis.

Symptoms include watery diarrhea, abdominal cramps, and gas.

4.1.3 SCHISTOSOMIASIS

Schistosomiasis is a chronic disease caused by parasitic worms. Symptoms include abdominal pain, diarrhea, blood in the stool, and fever. In severe cases, schistosomiasis can lead to liver damage, kidney failure, and bladder cancer.

4.2 SYMPTOMS AND CLINICAL MANIFESTATIONS

The symptoms of parasitic infections can vary widely, depending on the type of parasite, the location of the infection, and the1 individual's immune response. Common symptoms include:

Gastrointestinal symptoms: Diarrhea, constipation, abdominal pain, nausea, and vomiting.

Respiratory symptoms: Cough, shortness of breath, and wheezing.

Neurological symptoms: Headache, seizures, and cognitive impairment.

Skin symptoms: Rashes, itching, and skin lesions.

Systemic symptoms: Fever, fatigue, and weight loss.

In addition to acute symptoms, parasitic infections can have long-term consequences for human health.

4.3.1 CHRONIC INFLAMMATION

Chronic inflammation is a common feature of many parasitic infections. This can lead to tissue damage and an increased risk of developing chronic diseases, such as cancer and cardiovascular disease.

4.3.2 AUTOIMMUNE DISORDERS

Some parasitic infections have been linked to the development of autoimmune disorders, such as inflammatory bowel disease and rheumatoid arthritis. This may be due to the parasite's ability to mimic host antigens, triggering an autoimmune response.

4.4 CASE STUDIES: PARASITES AND MENTAL HEALTH

In recent years, researchers have begun to explore the link between parasitic infections and mental health disorders. Some studies have suggested that certain parasites may contribute to the development of conditions such as depression, anxiety, and schizophrenia.

By understanding the complex relationship between parasites and human health, we can develop effective strategies to prevent and treat parasitic infections and improve global health outcomes.

CHAPTER 5: THE INTERPLAY BETWEEN PARASITES AND THE HUMAN MICROBIOME

5.1 OVERVIEW OF THE HUMAN MICROBIOME

The human microbiome refers to the vast community of microorganisms, including bacteria, fungi, and viruses, that inhabit our bodies. These microorganisms play a crucial role in maintaining our health by aiding in digestion, producing essential vitamins, and protecting us from pathogens.

5.2 HOW PARASITES INFLUENCE MICROBIAL COMMUNITIES

Parasites can have a significant impact on the composition and function of the human microbiome. Some parasites, such as helminths, can directly compete with beneficial bacteria for nutrients, leading to alterations in the microbial community. Additionally, parasites can induce inflammation, which can further disrupt the delicate balance of the microbiome.

The human microbiome can play a crucial role in modulating the course of parasitic infections. A diverse and balanced microbiome can help to prevent colonization by pathogenic microorganisms, including parasites. Certain bacterial species have been shown to produce antimicrobial compounds that can inhibit the growth of parasites. Furthermore, the microbiota can influence the host's immune response, which can impact the severity of parasitic infections.

5.4 THERAPEUTIC IMPLICATIONS: PROBIOTICS AND ANTIPARASITIC TREATMENTS

The growing understanding of the interplay between parasites and the human microbiome has led to the development of new therapeutic approaches. Probiotics, which contain live microorganisms, have been shown to be effective in restoring the balance of the gut microbiota and may help to prevent or treat parasitic infections.

Antiparasitic drugs are used to treat a wide range of parasitic infections. However, the indiscriminate use of these drugs can lead to the development of drug-resistant parasites. To address this issue, researchers are exploring novel therapeutic approaches, such as the use of bacteriophages and other natural antimicrobial agents.

By understanding the complex relationship between parasites, the human microbiome, and the immune system, we can develop more effective strategies to prevent and treat parasitic infections and promote human health.

CHAPTER 6: EVOLUTION OF PARASITES AND HOSTS

6.1 COEVOLUTION OF PARASITES AND HUMAN HOSTS

The relationship between parasites and their hosts is a dynamic one, shaped by millions of years of coevolution. As parasites adapt to their hosts, hosts, in turn, evolve defenses to resist infection. This ongoing evolutionary arms race has led to the development of a diverse array of parasitic strategies and host defenses.

6.2 GENETIC ADAPTATIONS IN PARASITES

Parasites have evolved a variety of genetic adaptations to increase their fitness and transmission. These adaptations include:

Antigenic Variation: Rapidly changing surface antigens to evade the host's immune response.

Drug Resistance: Developing resistance to antiparasitic drugs, making treatment more challenging.

Enhanced Virulence: Increasing the severity of disease to maximize transmission.

6.3 THE EVOLUTIONARY ARMS RACE: HOST RESISTANCE VS. PARASITE VIRULENCE

The evolutionary arms race between parasites and hosts is a constant struggle. As parasites evolve new strategies to infect and exploit their hosts, hosts evolve counterstrategies to resist infection. This ongoing battle has led to the development of complex immune systems in many organisms, including humans.

6.4 INSIGHTS FROM PALEOPARASITOLOGY

Paleoparasitology, the study of ancient parasites, provides valuable insights into the coevolutionary history of parasites and humans. By examining the remains of ancient human populations, researchers can identify the parasites that afflicted our ancestors and learn about the strategies they used to survive and reproduce.

Understanding the evolutionary history of parasites can help us to develop more effective strategies to prevent and control parasitic infections. By studying the genetic adaptations of parasites, we can identify new drug targets and develop novel therapies. Additionally, by understanding the coevolutionary dynamics between parasites and hosts, we can gain insights into the emergence of new infectious diseases.

CHAPTER 7: DIAGNOSIS AND TREATMENT OF PARASITIC INFECTIONS

7.1 DIAGNOSTIC TECHNIQUES

Accurate and timely diagnosis of parasitic infections is crucial for effective treatment and prevention. A variety of diagnostic techniques are used to identify and diagnose parasitic infections:

7.1.1 MICROSCOPY

Microscopy remains a fundamental tool for diagnosing parasitic infections. By examining stool samples, blood smears, or tissue biopsies under a microscope, healthcare professionals can identify the presence of parasites or their eggs.

7.1.2 SEROLOGICAL TESTS

Serological tests detect antibodies produced by the body in response to a parasitic infection. These tests can be useful for diagnosing infections that are difficult to detect by microscopy, such as those caused by some protozoa.

7.1.3 MOLECULAR METHODS

Molecular methods, such as polymerase chain reaction (PCR), are highly sensitive and specific techniques that can detect the genetic material of parasites. These methods are particularly useful for diagnosing infections that are difficult to detect by other means, such as those caused by certain helminths and protozoa.

7.2 TREATMENT OPTIONS

The treatment of parasitic infections depends on the type of parasite and the severity of the infection.

7.2.1 ANTIPARASITIC MEDICATIONS

Antiparasitic medications, or anthelmintics, are used to kill or expel parasites from the body. These medications target specific stages of the parasite's life cycle and can be administered orally, topically, or intravenously.

7.2.2 VACCINATION STRATEGIES

Vaccination is an effective way to prevent parasitic infections. Vaccines work by stimulating the body's immune system to produce antibodies against specific parasites. While there are currently vaccines available for some parasitic diseases, such as malaria, the development of effective vaccines for other parasites remains a significant challenge.

One of the major challenges in treating parasitic infections is the emergence of drug resistance. As parasites are exposed to antiparasitic drugs, they can develop resistance mechanisms that allow them to survive and reproduce. This can lead to treatment failures and the spread of drug-resistant parasites.

Another challenge is the recurrence of infection. Many parasites have complex life cycles that involve multiple hosts. If all infected individuals in a community are not treated, the parasite can continue to circulate, leading to reinfection.

Additionally, some parasites can form dormant stages, which can reactivate and cause disease at a later time.

8.1 Global Burden of Parasitic Diseases

Parasitic diseases continue to pose a significant global health burden, particularly in low-income countries. They contribute to malnutrition, stunted growth, and cognitive impairment, especially in children. Moreover, parasitic infections can exacerbate other health problems and increase mortality rates.

8.2 STRATEGIES FOR PREVENTION

Effective prevention strategies are essential to control and eliminate parasitic diseases.

8.2.1 HYGIENE AND SANITATION

Improved Water Quality: Access to clean water and adequate sanitation facilities is crucial for preventing waterborne parasitic infections.

Proper Food Hygiene: Safe food handling practices, including thorough cooking and proper storage, can reduce the risk of foodborne parasitic infections.

Personal Hygiene: Regular handwashing with soap and water can help prevent the spread of many parasitic diseases, especially those transmitted through fecal-oral routes.

8.2.2 EDUCATION AND AWARENESS PROGRAMS

Public health education campaigns can raise awareness about the risks of parasitic infections and promote preventive measures. These programs should focus on:

Vector Control: Educating the public about the importance of vector control measures, such as using mosquito nets and insecticides.

Early Diagnosis and Treatment: Promoting early diagnosis and treatment of parasitic infections to prevent complications and reduce transmission.

8.3 POLICY IMPLICATIONS FOR GLOBAL HEALTH INITIATIVES

To effectively address the global burden of parasitic diseases, policymakers and international organizations must prioritize the following:

Increased Funding: Investing in research and development to develop new drugs, vaccines, and diagnostic tools.

Strengthening Health Systems: Improving access to healthcare services, especially in rural and underserved areas.

International Collaboration: Fostering international cooperation to share knowledge and resources.

Sustainable Development Goals: Integrating parasite control into broader development initiatives, such as poverty reduction and environmental sustainability.

8.4 CASE STUDIES: SUCCESSFUL ERADICATION PROGRAMS

Several successful eradication programs demonstrate the power of coordinated global efforts:

Dracunculiasis (Guinea Worm Disease): Through a concerted global effort, the incidence of dracunculiasis has been dramatically reduced.

Rinderpest: This devastating cattle disease was eradicated through a global vaccination campaign.

Smallpox: A highly contagious viral disease, smallpox was eradicated through a global vaccination program.

By learning from these successes and applying innovative strategies, we can work towards a future where parasitic diseases are no longer a major public health threat.

CHAPTER 9: FUTURE DIRECTIONS IN PARASITIC RESEARCH

9.1 EMERGING PARASITES AND NOVEL THREATS

The field of parasitology continues to evolve, with new and emerging parasites posing significant threats to human health. Factors such as climate change, globalization, and human migration can contribute to the emergence of new parasitic diseases. It is crucial to monitor these trends and develop effective strategies to prevent and control them.

9.2 ADVANCES IN RESEARCH METHODOLOGIES

Recent advancements in research methodologies have revolutionized our understanding of parasites and their interactions with hosts. These advancements include:

Genomics and Bioinformatics: Analyzing the genetic makeup of parasites can provide insights into their evolutionary history, virulence factors, and drug resistance mechanisms.

Proteomics: Studying the proteins expressed by parasites can help identify potential drug targets and vaccine antigens.

Metabolomics: Analyzing the metabolic profiles of parasites can reveal information about their energy metabolism, nutrient acquisition, and drug resistance.

9.3 INTERDISCIPLINARY APPROACHES TO UNDERSTANDING PARASITISM

A multidisciplinary approach is essential to fully understand the complex biology of parasites and the impact of parasitic infections on human health. By combining expertise from various fields, such as immunology, microbiology, genetics, and epidemiology, researchers can gain a more comprehensive understanding of these organisms.

9.4 THE ROLE OF TECHNOLOGY IN PARASITE CONTROL

Technological advancements have the potential to revolutionize parasite control. Some promising technologies include:

Nanotechnology: Developing nanomaterials for targeted drug delivery and diagnostic tools.

Biotechnology: Engineering genetically modified organisms to control parasite populations or produce therapeutic agents.

Artificial Intelligence: Using AI-powered tools to analyze large datasets, identify patterns, and predict outbreaks.

By embracing innovation and interdisciplinary collaboration, we can continue to make significant progress in the fight against parasitic diseases.

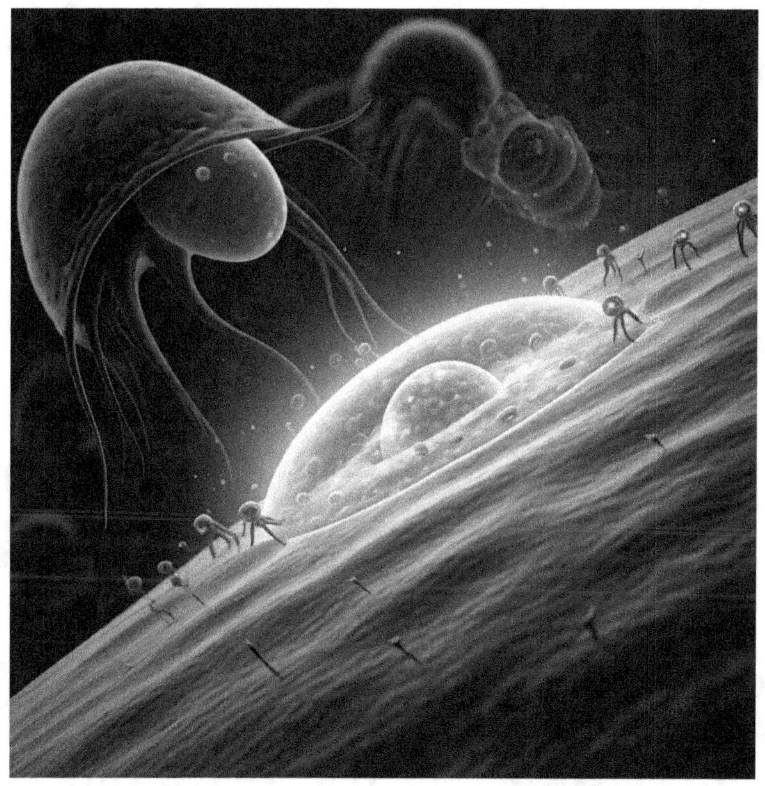

Throughout this book, we have explored the fascinating world of parasites, from their diverse forms and complex life cycles to their profound impact on human health and society. We have examined the intricate interplay between parasites and their hosts, the mechanisms of parasite transmission, and the strategies they employ to evade the immune system.

We have also delved into the neurobiological effects of parasitic infections, the role of the microbiome in modulating host-parasite interactions, and the evolutionary arms race between parasites and their hosts. Additionally, we have discussed the challenges associated with diagnosing and treating parasitic infections, as well as the importance of preventive measures and public health initiatives.

THE ONGOING RELATIONSHIP BETWEEN HUMANS AND PARASITES

The relationship between humans and parasites is a dynamic one that has shaped the course of human history. As our understanding of these organisms grows, so too does our ability to combat the diseases they cause. However, the emergence of new parasites and the development of drug resistance continue to pose significant challenges.

CALL TO ACTION: EDUCATION, RESEARCH, AND POLICY

To address these challenges, it is crucial to prioritize education, research, and policy initiatives. By raising awareness about parasitic infections and promoting preventive measures, we can reduce the burden of these diseases. Continued investment in research is essential to develop new diagnostic tools, vaccines, and treatments. Additionally, strong public health policies are needed to ensure access to healthcare, improve sanitation, and promote sustainable development.

By working together, we can break the cycle of parasitic infections and create a healthier future for all.

1. THE IMPACT OF MALARIA IN SUB-SAHARAN AFRICA

Malaria, a mosquito-borne disease caused by Plasmodium parasites, remains a major public health problem in Sub-Saharan Africa. The disease has a profound impact on individuals, communities, and economies.

KEY IMPACTS:

High Morbidity and Mortality: Malaria causes significant morbidity and mortality, particularly among young children and pregnant women.

Economic Burden: The disease reduces productivity, increases healthcare costs, and hinders economic development.

Social Disruption: Malaria can disrupt education, social activities, and family life.

Control and Prevention Strategies:

Vector Control: Using insecticide-treated nets, indoor residual spraying, and larvicides to reduce mosquito populations.

Drug Treatment: Administering effective antimalarial drugs to treat infected individuals.

Vaccine Development: Ongoing research to develop a highly effective malaria vaccine.

Community Engagement: Empowering communities to take ownership of malaria prevention and control efforts.

2. Toxoplasmosis and Its Effects on Human Behavior

Toxoplasma gondii is a parasite that can infect a wide range of animals, including humans. While most infections are asymptomatic, in some cases, it can cause serious health problems, particularly in immunocompromised individuals.

BEHAVIORAL MANIPULATION:

One of the most intriguing aspects of Toxoplasma gondii is its ability to manipulate the behavior of its infected hosts. In rodents, the parasite can alter their behavior, making them more likely to be preyed upon by cats, the definitive host for the parasite. This manipulation is thought to be mediated by changes in the host's brain chemistry.

PUBLIC HEALTH IMPLICATIONS:

While most infections are mild, Toxoplasma gondii can cause severe illness in pregnant women and immunocompromised individuals. It is important to practice good hygiene, especially when handling raw meat or cat litter, to reduce the risk of infection.

3. Schistosomiasis and Economic Burden in Endemic Regions

Schistosomiasis, a waterborne parasitic disease caused by Schistosoma worms, affects millions of people worldwide, primarily in sub-Saharan Africa, South America, and parts of Asia.

ECONOMIC IMPACT:

Schistosomiasis can have a significant economic impact on endemic regions. The disease can lead to reduced productivity, increased healthcare costs, and lower educational attainment.

CONTROL AND PREVENTION STRATEGIES:

Praziquantel Treatment: Mass drug administration with praziquantel can effectively control the spread of schistosomiasis.

Improved Sanitation: Access to safe water and sanitation facilities can reduce exposure to the parasite.

Snail Control: Reducing the population of snails, which serve as intermediate hosts for the parasite, can help to control the spread of the disease.

Health Education: Raising awareness about the disease and promoting preventive measures can help reduce transmission.

By understanding the complex biology, epidemiology, and impact of these parasitic diseases, we can develop effective strategies to control and eliminate them.

Overview of Laboratory Techniques

Laboratory techniques are essential for the study of parasites. Some of the most common techniques include:

MICROSCOPY:

Light microscopy: Used to examine the morphology of parasites, including their size, shape, and internal structures.

Electron microscopy: Provides high-resolution images of parasite ultrastructure, revealing details of cell organelles and surface features.

PARASITOLOGICAL EXAMINATION:

Stool examination: Used to detect intestinal parasites and their eggs.

Blood smear examination: Used to detect blood parasites, such as malaria parasites.

Tissue biopsy: Used to examine tissues for the presence of parasites.

Polymerase Chain Reaction (PCR): A powerful technique for detecting and identifying parasites based on their DNA or RNA.

DNA sequencing: Used to determine the genetic sequence of parasites, which can help to identify new species and track the spread of drug resistance.

Enzyme-linked immunosorbent assay (ELISA): Used to detect antibodies against parasites in the blood of infected individuals.

Immunofluorescence assay: Used to visualize parasites in tissues or cells.

Field studies are essential for understanding the epidemiology of parasitic infections and for evaluating the effectiveness of control programs. Key epidemiological approaches include:

Cross-sectional studies: Used to determine the prevalence of infection in a population at a specific point in time.

Cohort studies: Used to track the incidence of disease over time in a defined population.

Case-control studies: Used to identify risk factors for infection by comparing cases of disease with controls.

Ethical Considerations in Parasitological Research

Ethical considerations are paramount in parasitological research, especially when involving human subjects. Key ethical principles include:

Informed consent: Participants should be fully informed about the study and its potential risks and benefits before providing consent.

Minimizing harm: Researchers should take all necessary steps to minimize harm to participants, including physical and psychological harm.

Confidentiality: Participant data should be kept confidential and protected from unauthorized access.

Animal welfare: When using animals in research, researchers must adhere to ethical guidelines to ensure their well-being.

Benefit-risk ratio: The potential benefits of the research must outweigh the risks to participants.

By adhering to these ethical principles, researchers can ensure that their work is conducted responsibly and ethically.

Recommended Books

Parasitology by K.D. Murrell: A comprehensive textbook covering the biology, epidemiology, and control of parasitic diseases.

The Parasite's Tale: A Microbial World Inside Us by Kathleen McAuliffe: A fascinating exploration of the intricate relationship between humans and parasites.

Principles of Tropical Medicine and Parasitology by Melvin E. Wilson and Anthony O.C. Orengo: A classic textbook covering the diagnosis, treatment, and prevention of tropical diseases.

RECOMMENDED JOURNALS

Parasitology

International Journal for Parasitology

Trends in Parasitology

The American Journal of Tropical Medicine and Hygiene

PLoS Neglected Tropical Diseases

Websites

Centers for Disease Control and Prevention (CDC): Provides information on parasitic diseases, prevention, and control.

World Health Organization (WHO): Offers global health information and statistics on parasitic diseases.

American Society of Tropical Medicine and Hygiene (ASTMH): A professional society dedicated to advancing tropical medicine and parasitology.

ORGANIZATIONS FOCUSED ON PARASITOLOGY AND GLOBAL HEALTH

World Health Organization (WHO): A specialized agency of the United Nations responsible for international public health.

Centers for Disease Control and Prevention (CDC):1 A federal agency responsible for protecting public health and safety.

Wellcome Trust: A global charitable foundation supporting scientific research to improve health.

Drugs for Neglected Diseases initiative (DNDi): A non-profit organization developing new treatments for neglected tropical diseases.

By exploring these resources, you can delve deeper into the fascinating world of parasitology and contribute to the ongoing efforts to combat parasitic diseases.

THE HUMAN MICROBIOME AND PARASITES

The human microbiome plays a critical role in maintaining health and preventing disease. However, imbalances in the microbiome can create opportunities for parasites to colonize the gut and cause infection. Understanding the complex interactions between the microbiome and parasites is essential for developing effective strategies to prevent and treat parasitic diseases.

ETHICAL CONSIDERATIONS IN PARASITE RESEARCH

Ethical considerations are paramount in parasitological research, particularly when involving human subjects. Researchers must adhere to strict ethical guidelines to ensure the safety and well-being of participants. This includes obtaining informed consent, minimizing harm, and protecting privacy.

THE FUTURE OF PARASITE CONTROL

As the world faces new challenges, such as climate change and globalization, the threat of emerging and re-emerging parasitic diseases is increasing. To address these challenges, it is crucial to invest in research and development, strengthen public health infrastructure, and promote international cooperation. By working together, we can build a healthier future and reduce the burden of parasitic diseases.

PERSONALITY CHANGES ASSOCIATED WITH PARASITE INFECTION

While the impact of parasites on human health is often associated with physical symptoms, some parasites can also influence human behavior and cognition.1 One of the most well-studied examples is Toxoplasma gondii.2

TOXOPLASMA GONDII AND BEHAVIORAL CHANGES

Toxoplasma gondii is a parasite commonly found in cats.3 Humans can become infected by consuming undercooked meat or through contact with cat feces.4 While most infections are asymptomatic, the parasite can form cysts in the brain, potentially leading to behavioral changes.5

Some studies have linked Toxoplasma gondii infection to:

Increased risk-taking behavior: Infected individuals may exhibit more impulsive and reckless behavior.6

Altered personality traits: Changes in personality, such as increased suspicion, jealousy, and anxiety.

Neuropsychiatric disorders: Some researchers suggest a link between Toxoplasma gondii infection and conditions like schizophrenia and bipolar disorder.7

It's important to note that the extent of these effects can vary widely among individuals. Factors such as the individual's immune system, genetic predisposition, and overall health can influence the severity of symptoms.

While Toxoplasma gondii is the most well-studied parasite linked to behavioral changes, other parasites may also have subtle effects on human behavior and cognition. Further research is needed to fully understand the mechanisms underlying these effects and to develop strategies to mitigate their impact.

qualified healthcare provider with any questions you may have regarding a medical condition.2

While this book strives to provide accurate and up-to-date information about parasitology, it is important to note that scientific knowledge and medical practices are continually evolving. The information presented here should not be considered as a substitute for professional medical advice.

If you have concerns about your health or suspect a parasitic infection, please consult with a qualified healthcare professional. The information provided in this book is for general knowledge and educational purposes only.

IT IS RECOMMENDED TO CONSULT WITH HEALTHCARE PROFESSIONALS FOR PERSONALIZED ADVICE AND DIAGNOSIS. THE CONTENT OF THIS BOOK IS INTENDED FOR GENERAL KNOWLEDGE AND INFORMATIONAL PURPOSES ONLY, AND SHOULD NOT BE CONSIDERED AS A SUBSTITUTE FOR PROFESSIONAL MEDICAL ADVICE.